HOW-TO CIALIS GUIDE

Understanding its Role in Treating ED and BPD

DR. CRAIG MIRACLE

Table of Contents

CHAPTER ONE 4

   Understanding Cialis 4

Alternatives to Cialis 10

Potential Side Effects of Cialis 17

Interactions with other medications 21

Benefits of using Cialis 26

CHAPTER TWO 31

   Lifestyle changes to support Cialis 31

Dosage and Administration 35

Things you know before taking Cialis 39

When to see a doctor 43

Errors to avoid 45

THE END 50

CHAPTER ONE
Understanding Cialis

Cialis also known as tadalafil is a medication used for treating erectile dysfunction in both men and women, but especially in men. This powerful medication comes in tablet form and works by causing blood to flow to the penis thereby ensuring a firm and long-lasting erection for sexual intercourse.

The effect of Cialis can last between the duration of 3-6 hours, and it is best recommended to take Cialis 30-60 minutes before the sexual activity as it becomes effective after 30 minutes of usage.

There is no general recommendation in terms of the required dosage to take as this depends largely on the individual's level of tolerance for the medication. Though powerful and undoubtedly effective, there are other ways to fight erectile dysfunction without using Cialis. For instance, engaging in regular physical exercises such as running, swimming, and skiing can help enhance the flow of the body throughout the body including the penile region. Also, eating natural feeds such as fruits, vegetables, nuts, and legumes can help fight off erectile dysfunction in men.

Alternatives to Cialis

Without undermining the effectiveness of

Cialis, it is also safe and essential to note the alternatives to this medication. There are several alternatives to Cialis for the treatment of erectile dysfunction and one of them is Cialis; which provides an even longer period of erection for sexual intercourse. Another effective Cialis alternative that has lesser risks of side effects and lasts longer than Cialis is Levitra.

Furthermore, there are many other natural remedies, supplements, medications, and lifestyle changes that could be adopted to help achieve and maintain a firm erection for sexual activities.

Medications such as vardenafil and sildenafil can also be used to solve erectile dysfunction.

Engaging in regular exercises such as swimming, running,

and skiing; in addition to adopting lifestyle changes that prohibit incessant smoking and intake of alcohol can go a long way in helping you achieve and maintain a firm and long-lasting erection for sexual intercourse.

Potential Side Effects of Cialis

Though effective and very well tolerated, this medication can exhibit severely damaging side effects in the long term if not properly used. The most common side effects of Cialis are; reddening of the facial skin, vision problems, diarrhea, and a blocked nose. An overuse or misuse of Cialis could also lead to troubling long-term side effects such as painful erections and other disturbing allergic reactions. Patients with a medical history of erectile dysfunction or on other medications are more exposed to complicated side effects. Hence, it is best advised to consult your medical doctor for guidance, and endeavor to report any experienced side effects during usage to your medical doctor for better treatment.

Interactions with other medications

Taking Cialis in the same period as other medications, natural remedies or supplements would render either or both of the medications ineffective and result to severely damaging side-effects. Hence, the need to consult a doctor or pharmacist about your condition should be underlined and taken seriously.

Drugs such as nitrate should not be combined with Cialis as a combination of the two would lead to a drastic decrease in blood pressure.

Avoid the intake of alcohol or grapefruit juice during the course of Cialis usage as both naturally decrease blood pressure.

Some medications such as protease are capable of enhancing

the levels of Cialis in your bloodstream, living you susceptible to side effects. This medication should not be taken in the same period as Cialis.

Benefits of using Cialis

There are many benefits that come with using this powerful and effective medication. The primary goal of Cialis is to cure erectile dysfunction in men. It works by enhancing the flow of blood to various parts of the body such as the penis; making it possible to achieve and maintain a firm and long-lasting erection for sexual activity. A firm and long-lasting erection guarantees a satisfied sexual experience for the couple and this increases self-confidence in the man and improves the intimacy in a relationship. The increased flow of blood to the brain improves cognitive functionality, making it easy to learn.

This increased flow of blood throughout the body allows for a regulation of the body's glucose level;

hence minimizing the occurrence of diabetes. It also helps to reduce the occurrence of heart attacks, and stroke and brings relief to back pains.

CHAPTER TWO

Lifestyle changes to support Cialis

Apart from treating erectile dysfunction medically with Cialis, there are certain lifestyles that can be adopted to improve, support, and maintain erectile health. Engaging in regular physical exercises can help improve cardiovascular issues and cause regular and increased flow of blood to the penis and the rest of the body. Engaging in mental exercises such as yoga, and meditation can help relieve the mind and body of stress, anxiety, and depression, and this can in turn boost the sexual health of a man. Excessive smoking and intake of alcohol are detrimental to one's sexual life; hence it is best advised to restrain from this choice of lifestyle to improve, support, and maintain erectile health.

Dosage and Administration

It is best to consult a medical doctor especially when it comes to the dosage and administration of Cialis. Nevertheless, Cialis comes in tablet form with dosages between 25mg to 100mg. It is best advised to start your dosage with 50mg and to be taken an hour before any sexual intercourse.

Taking more than the maximum dosage of 100mg in a 24-hour period could result in allergic reactions and other painful sensations in the penis. Endeavor to seek the help of a healthcare professional if you experience any disturbing reactions or side effects.

Things you know before taking Cialis

Cialis is an effective way of treating

erectile dysfunction in men. However, there are certain things you should know before considering the usage of the medication. Cialis does not interact well with alcohol. Its duration of effectiveness varies for every individual. Though, the most common duration is between 3-5 hours. It can also improve cardiovascular and cognitive functions. The intake of Cialis helps the body to regulate its glucose level. Those who use Cialis can engage in regular physical exercises without the risk of heart attacks or other cardiovascular issues.

When to see a doctor

Excessive use of Cialis could result in painful erections in the penis and other disturbing allergic reactions. Seek the guidance of your doctor for the proper usage of this medication for maximum effectiveness. Also, ensure to tell your pharmacist or doctor if you experience any of the aforementioned side effects of using Cialis.

Errors to avoid

The effectiveness of this medication is dependent on the usage of it. Though effective in curing erectile dysfunction, there are certain errors to avoid and precautionary measures to adhere to in order to get the effectiveness of this medication and reduce the chances of experiencing adverse side effects. Avoid the intake of alcohol while using

Cialis to treat erectile dysfunction. Do not take more than the dosage prescribed by your pharmacist or doctor. Talk to your doctor about other medications you might be taking to

cure   erectile
dysfunction.

THE END

www.ingramcontent.com/pod-product-compliance
Lightning Source LLC
Chambersburg PA
CBHW072019230526
45479CB00008B/303